DISEASE OUTBREAK MANAGEMENT
Hospital Administrators' Perspective

"Nise Dominus Frusta"

"Without God We can Do Nothing"

DISEASE OUTBREAK MANAGEMENT
Hospital Administrators' Perspective

Shakti Kumar Gupta
MBBS MHA (AIIMS) FNAMS FIHE FAHA FIMSA
Head
Department of Hospital Administration
Medical Superintendent
All India Institute of Medical Sciences
Dr Rajendra Prasad Centre for Ophthalmic Sciences and
Jai Prakash Narayan Apex Trauma Centre
New Delhi, India

Sunil Kant
MBBS DCE DCA MBA MHA
Army Medical Corps

Jitendra Kumar Sharma
PhD MBA PGHEP PGCQM PGHM LSM (Harvard School)
Clinical Faculty
University of Adelaide, Australia

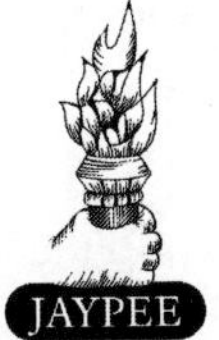

JAYPEE BROTHERS MEDICAL PUBLISHERS
The Health Sciences Publisher
New Delhi | London

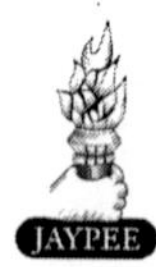

Jaypee Brothers Medical Publishers (P) Ltd

Headquarters
EMCA House
23/23-B, Ansari Road, Daryaganj
New Delhi 110 002, India
Landline: +91-11-23272143, +91-11-23272703
+91-11-23282021, +91-11-23245672
E-mail: jaypee@jaypeebrothers.com

Corporate Office
4838/24, Ansari Road, Daryaganj
New Delhi 110 002, India
Phone: +91-11-43574357
Fax: +91-11-43574314
E-mail: jaypee@jaypeebrothers.com

Overseas Office
J.P. Medical Ltd
83 Victoria Street, London
SW1H 0HW (UK)
Phone: +44 20 3170 8910
E-mail: info@jpmedpub.com

EU GPSR Authorised Representative
Logos Europe, 9 rue Nicolas Poussin
17000, La Rochelle, France
Phone: +33 (0) 6 67 93 73 78
E-mail: contact@logoseurope.eu

Website: www.jaypeebrothers.com
Website: www.jaypeedigital.com

© 2013, Authors

All rights reserved. No part of this book may be reproduced in any form or by any means without the prior permission of the publisher.

Inquiries for bulk sales may be solicited at: jaypee@jaypeebrothers.com

This book has been published in good faith that the contents provided by the authors contained herein are original, and is intended for educational purposes only. While every effort is made to ensure accuracy of information, the publisher and the authors specifically disclaim any damage, liability, or loss incurred, directly or indirectly, from the use or application of any of the contents of this work. If not specifically stated, all figures and tables are courtesy of the authors.

Disease Outbreak Management: Hospital Administrators' Perspective

First Edition: **2013**

Reprint: **2026**

ISBN 978-93-5025-990-0

Printed at: Samrat Offset Pvt. Ltd.

Dedicated to

The extraordinary efforts of all those
who have contributed in the mitigation of adverse
events and prevention of disease outbreaks

Preface

Disease outbreaks are inevitable and often unpredictable events. Early identification of the cause and the source of the outbreak can limit the spread of the outbreak. A rapid outbreak response can reduce morbidity, mortality and disability by promoting appropriate, evidence-based and prompt case management. An outbreak plan provides guidance on managing outbreaks of communicable disease in health facilities. It is intended to ensure prompt action to recognize an outbreak of communicable disease, eliminate the source, stop further spread, prevent recurrence, and ensure effective communication between all concerned. The key to a good response is adequate planning, multistage assessment and comprehensive response. The book details the various issues that would emerge in a healthcare institution while responding to a disease outbreak. It is a known fact that in times of a disease outbreak, health systems are under stress and resources far overstretched. Prioritizing the issues, pre-set strategy, standardized protocols, and methodology to assess the preparedness, are some of the key factors which are essential and have been dealt with in the book.

The role of hospital administrators in handling a disease outbreak situation has been elaborated. While the sudden increase in patient load tends to create barriers on the day-to-day functioning of the hospitals, the control and response to the disease becomes challenging. Comprehensive understanding of the role that hospital administrators have to assume during disease outbreaks should be specified for effective and efficient management of disease outbreaks which could lead to a larger community benefit and a greater health protection. A checklist has been developed utilizing which the hospitals can rate and assess their preparedness status. Gaps if any, in planning and implementation process may accordingly be reduced/eliminated. The book is intended for hospital administrators, healthcare providers, medical superintendents and clinico-managerial executives for efficient management of outbreak response. It will be of immense benefit to healthcare institutions and hospitals in strengthening their capacity and assuring multifocal strategy while managing situations arising out of a disease outbreak. It will also aid policy-makers in enunciating/amending/augmenting operational and strategic policies related to disease outbreak management.

Authors

Contents

Abbreviations

ADR	Adverse Drug Reaction
AIDS	Acquired Immunodeficiency Syndrome
BMWM	Bio-Medical Waste Management
BSNL	Bharat Sanchar Nigam Limited
CBRN	Chemical, Biological, Radiological, and Nuclear
CDC	Center for Disease Control
CSSD	Central Sterile Supply Department
DEPT	Department
EI	Epidemic Intelligence
HIV	Human Immunodeficiency Virus
HOCT	Hospital Outbreak Control Team
ICT	Infection Control Team
IDSP	Integrated Disease Surveillance Project
IHR	International Health Regulations
MII	Malaria Institute of India
MTNL	Mahanagar Telephone Nigam Limited
NAMP	National Anti-Malaria Programme
NDMA	National Disaster Management Authority
NICD	National Institute of Communicable Diseases
NMEP	National Malaria Eradication Programme
OCT	Outbreak Control Team
OPD	Outpatient Department
PCR	Polymerase Chain Reaction
PFGE	Pulsed Field Gel Electrophoresis
PPE	Personal Protective Equipment
PV	Pharmacovigilance
QRT	Quick Reaction Team
RT-PCR	Reverse Transcriptase-Polymerase Chain Reaction
RRT	Rapid Response Team
SARS	Severe Acute Respiratory Syndrome
SARS-CV	Severe Acute Respiratory Syndrome-Corona Virus

SOCO	Single Overriding Communication Objective
SOPs	Standing Operating Procedures
STEC	Shiga Toxin Producing *Escherichia coli*
UTs	Union Territories
VAP	Ventilator-associated Pneumonia
VISA	Vancomycin Intermediate *Staphylococcus aureus*
VRSA	Vancomycin Respiratory *Staphylococcus aureus*
WHO	World Health Organization

CHAPTER

Disease Outbreak Management: An Overview

INTRODUCTION

It is an accepted fact that in improvement of healthcare status of a community preventive measures are of more significance than curative remedies. Diseases outbreaks often cause public health emergencies with resultant increased morbidity and mortality. In India, many communicable diseases are endemic. These often have seasonal and cyclic trends and have potential to cause outbreaks. Disease outbreaks cannot always be predicted or prevented, however, timely investigation and application of specific control measures may limit the spread of the outbreak and prevent deaths.

A planned healthcare delivery, or for that matter, even an immunization program needs a different approach than a sudden outburst of disease something which is commonly known as an outbreak. The need for a preordained guideline regarding disease outbreak management is an essential requirement. There is also a need for a compact assessment tool which will facilitate the healthcare institutions to assess their preparedness for handling an outbreak. Guidelines would also equip the healthcare providers in strategic provisioning of healthcare resources.

There are many organizations and institutions that participate and contribute in limiting, restricting and terminating disease outbreak. The role of a healthcare institution becomes an area of special importance. The healthcare institution needs to respond in accordance with the National and International accepted norms to manage the outbreak. Hospital Administrators need to guide, direct, motivate, train and analyze operational and strategic imperatives for managing the disease outbreaks.

DEFINITIONS

World Health Organization defines disease outbreak as occurrence of disease in excess than what would normally be expected in a defined community, geographical area or season. An outbreak may occur in a restricted geographical area, or may extend over several countries. It may last for few days or weeks or several years.

A single case of communicable disease long absent from a population or caused by an infective agent not previously recognized in that community or area, or the emergence of a previously unknown disease, may also constitute an outbreak and should be reported and investigated.

Last's Dictionary of Epidemiology defines outbreak as "An epidemic limited to a localized increase in the incidence of a disease". An outbreak is limited or localized to a village, town or closed institution. However, the magnitude could involve wider geographical areas even beyond one district, where it may assume the dimension of an epidemic. Center disease control (CDC) uses the term "outbreak" synonymous with "epidemic". Public health officials often use the term "outbreak" so as to avoid panic since the term epidemic may denote grave and beyond control.

Epidemic/Disease outbreak indicate a "higher than normal" element. In the practical sense, at the public health level the term "outbreak" is used when the health of human or animal population is impacted necessitating investigation. The factors which determine the need to proceed with investigation are:

- Cost and effort of the investigation.
- Determination of resource priority.
- Magnitude of the illness.

CLASSIFICATION OF OUTBREAKS

Outbreaks are usually classified into categories of Endemic, Epidemic and Pandemic.

Endemic

It is derived from Greak word *en* meaning in or within and *demos* meaning people. In epidemiology, an infection is said to be endemic in a population when that infection is maintained in the population without the need for external inputs. For an infection that relies on person-to-person transmission, to be endemic, each person who becomes infected with the disease must transmit it on to one other person on an average, assuming a completely susceptible population that means that the basic reproduction number (R_0) of the infection must equal 1. In a population with some immune individuals, the basic reproduction number multiplied by the proportion of susceptible individuals in the population (S) must be 1. This takes account of the probability of each individual, to whom the disease may be transmitted actually being susceptible to it, effectively discounting the immune sector of the population. For the disease to be in an endemic steady state,

$$R_0 \times S = 1$$

The infection neither terminates nor do the numbers of infected people increase exponentially but remains in an endemic steady state, e.g. malaria is endemic in North-Eastern States of India.

Epidemic

It is derived from Greek word *epi* meaning upon or above and *demos* meaning people. In epidemiology, an epidemic, occurs when new cases of a certain disease, in a given human population, and during a given period, substantially exceed what is expected based on recent experience. The disease may be communicable or noncommunicable. Examples of noncommunicable epidemics are cancer, heart disease. An epidemic may be restricted to one locale, more general, or even global, in which case it is called a pandemic. A few cases of a very rare disease may be classified as an epidemic, while many cases of a common disease (such as the common cold) would not.

Pandemic

It is derived from Greek word *pan* meaning all and *demos* meaning people. A pandemic is an epidemic of infectious disease that is spreading through human populations across a large region; for instance a continent, or even worldwide. A widespread endemic disease that is stable in terms of how many people are getting sick from it is not a pandemic. Further, flu pandemics exclude seasonal flu, unless the flu of the season is a pandemic. Throughout history, there have been a number of pandemics, such as smallpox and tuberculosis. More recent pandemics include the HIV pandemic and the 2009 flu pandemic. The occurrence of an epidemic always signals some significant shift in the existing balance between the agent, host and environment. It calls for a prompt and thorough investigation of the cases to identify the factor(s) responsible and to guide in advocating control measures to prevent further spread. Emergencies caused by epidemics remain one of the most important challenges to National Health Administrations.

An outbreak thus is any form of uncontrolled or controlled spread of disease which could trigger health hazard and adversely affect health indicators in a community.

CHAPTER

Role of Healthcare Institutions

WHEN AND HOW TO RESPOND?

A disease outbreak not only disrupts the normal flow of life in a community but also places hospital authorities, health agencies, district and general hospitals and medical college hospitals to a much increased activity load. It often stretches the activity to much beyond its maximum handling capacity. During an outbreak, the market price of required healthcare resources may escalate as occurred in case of facemasks during the H_1N_1 outbreak. This may result in a resource crunch and adversely affect resource distribution. A disease outbreak almost always is a constraint on healthcare resources.

The healthcare institutions should respond positively, adequately and energetically to the multiple challenges. A planned, synchronized and scientific approach is required. The factors according to which the action plan is to be made could be grouped under the following categories:

- When there are reports of unusual disease cases.
- Patients appear in hospital emergency departments, clinics, and primary care facilities in a much greater number than expected or suggested by previous years' trends.
- Increased hospital admissions with similar/related or secondary manifestations.
- Unusual deaths that might be caused by infectious diseases.
- Increase in number of reported sick calls from employers and schools.
- Increase in sales of over-the-counter medications.
- Increase in the number of ambulance calls.
- Increase in calls to healthcare hotlines.
- Information from veterinary disease reporting networks.
- International epidemiological information.

When one or more of the events mentioned above occurs healthcare institutions should take precautionary measures of a likely outbreak and take appropriate preventive, diagnostic and therapeutic actions.

DISEASE OUTBREAK MANAGEMENT PLAN

Define the Scope of the Outbreak

Once an outbreak has been identified and a case definition for that outbreak developed, investigators should define the scope of the outbreak. To do this, investigators should:

- Verify the diagnosis.
- Search for additional cases.

Verification of the Diagnosis

- If laboratory testing has already been performed, confirm that the laboratory results have been reported correctly.
- If laboratory testing has not been performed, collect clinical specimens for
  - Laboratory testing.
  - Encourage those who are ill to visit a physician, if not already done.

Search for Additional Cases

Depending on the outbreak and resources, the following activities can assist in searching for additional cases:

- Contact local physicians to notify them of the outbreak and request that specimens be collected from patients who may be a case in the outbreak. This can be done by phone, fax, or email. However, patient's right to privacy must be respected and individual specific information should be coded before recording.
- Conduct chart reviews at hospital emergency departments or physicians' offices for patients that may fit the case definition. These patients may not have previously been identified as part of the outbreak.
- Maintain frequent contact with local laboratories for any specimen's positive for the causative agent (if known) in the outbreak. This will reduce delay, in reporting of cases.

- Notify district health authorities and request information on related cases.
- Determine if other groups with the same exposure, suspected as the source of the outbreak, also experienced similar illness.
- When necessary, use public information avenues to notify the public of the outbreak and to invite those who may be a case to come forward.
- The relative emphasis on various components in a disease outbreak management is shown in Figure 2.1.

Disease agent		Outbreak source and transmission mechanism	
		Known	Unknown
	Known	Investigation + Control +++	Investigation +++ Control +
	Unknown	Investigation +++ Control +++	Investigation +++ Control +

(*Source:* Adopted from Goodman)

Notes: +++ high emphasis should be placed on this stage of outbreak management + low (or less) emphasis should be placed on this stage of outbreak management

Fig. 2.1: Relative emphasis of investigation and response during outbreak management, as influenced by levels of certainty about disease agent, source and transmission mechanism.

Investigation of Epidemic

The objectives of an epidemic investigation include assessing the magnitude of the epidemic outbreak, determining the conditions responsible, identifying the source(s) of infection, if any, and mode of transmission, and to make recommendations so as to prevent its recurrence. Epidemiological investigation is more than the collected established facts. It includes their orderly arrangement of data, chain of inference, which extend beyond just direct observation. A summary of the essential steps in management of an epidemic is given in Box 2.1.

At times the steps enumerated may be required to be followed concurrently rather than sequentially.

Box 2.1: Steps in disease outbreak management

- Provisional diagnosis and development of case definition.
- Establish a case definition (clinical and/or microbiological).
- Confirm existence of an epidemic.
- Line listing of cases. Patient, place and time of occurrence and infection details.
- Management of cases, including appropriate isolation or cohorting of infected cases.
- Community survey for further case finding.
- Appropriate entomological and environmental investigations.
- Laboratory investigations.
- *Data Analysis* – This includes:
  - Place and person analysis by maps and table formulation.
  - Time analysis by number of cases and time graph.
- Formulation of hypothesis should include characteristics of affected population, causes of disease, mode of transmission incubation period and likely cause of outbreak.
- Institution of control measures.
- Monitor control measures by continued surveillance for disease.
- *Report* – To include:
  - Interim report.
  - Final report.
- Testing of hypothesis.
- Declaration that the outbreak is over (After no new case in a period twice the incubation period of the disease).
- Evaluation of outbreak management.
- Documentation and sharing of lessons learnt.
- Determine, if any, changes are requested in policy/procedures.

Steps in Investigation

Important details of some of the steps are given below:

Verification of Diagnosis

Though laboratory confirmation of diagnosis is ideal a clinical examination of a sample of cases will also suffice for which use of rapid test kits should be explored. Details of epidemiological parameters should also be utilized for confirmation of diagnosis. Patients signs/symptoms, movement and contact history should be recorded.

Confirmation of Epidemic

The disease frequency of previous years (generally three) is compared. An epidemic is said to exist when the number of cases (observed frequency) is in excess of the expected frequency for that population, based on past experience. In statistical terms, limit of two standard errors from the endemic occurrence is used to define the epidemic threshold. A detailed and current map of the area and population census will be beneficial in further investigating the outbreak.

Medical Survey

Medical survey should be carried out to identify actual/potential patients. Information from patients and medical practitioners should also be incorporated in order to get a comprehensive situational analysis. This should be followed by:

- *Line listing of cases:* A line list is a serial, chronological listing of all the known cases. The details of cases should include name, age, sex, address (both residential and work place), main symptoms, time of onset of symptoms, details of healthcare facility where reported. A proper line listing helps in definitions of the disease, understanding disease transmission/dynamics and in delineating the population at risk. Case definition based on clinical and/or microbiological parameters should be developed and finalized so as to ensure the cases are appropriately identified and managed. The case may be categorized into definite, probable and suspect.
- *Epidemiological case sheet:* It includes details related to the patient such as name, age, sex, occupation, social class, travel, history of previous exposure, time of onset of disease, signs and symptoms of illness, personal contacts at home, work place, school and other places, immunization status, social interactions, history of attendance at large gatherings, food consumed, group travelling; visits out of the community, history of receiving injections or blood products. The epidemiological case sheet is also known as "case interview form".

- *Epidemiological description:* This is essential for developing hypothesis regarding various possible sources of exposures that may have caused the outbreak The cases should be described by time, place and person. The description should include:
  - *Estimating the attack rates:*

    i.e. $\frac{\text{Total case}}{\text{Population defined to be at risk}}$
  - *Describing the clinical-epidemiological profile*: This includes the details of the clinical presentation and also the number of fatalities.
  - *Cases description:* This would have details such as age groups, sex, occupation. In epidemics of gastroenteritis places where food was eaten, sources of drinking water and potential reasons for any household contamination should also be included.
  - *Describing the epidemic according to time* (Epidemic curve): A curve may be drawn with attack rate/actual number of cases on Y-axis and the unit of time along X-axis.
  - *Describing the epidemic according to place:* Spot maps should be made in which the frequency of disease is shown by colored dots.
  - *Describing the environment conditions before and during the outbreak:* Correlating these with line listing and person place and time distribution may indicate possible causes of the outbreak.

Epidemic Curve

The epidemic curve is a graphic representation of the distribution of cases by the time of onset. The shape of the epidemic curve may suggest a single point source, ongoing transmission or an intermittent source.

Plotting of disease accordingly to short time intervals may depict early warning signs of an epidemic. If the time period while plotting such short term fluctuations is one when an epidemic is actually occurring the line diagram or the histogram depicting it is called the epidemic curve. The recommended time interval along the X-axis should be a period which is

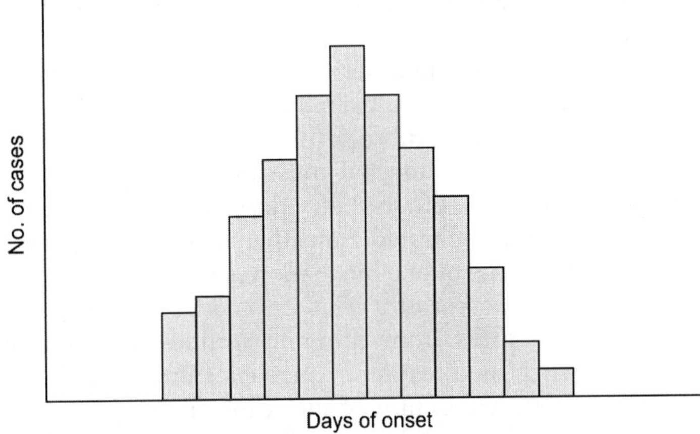

Fig. 2.2: Point source histogram

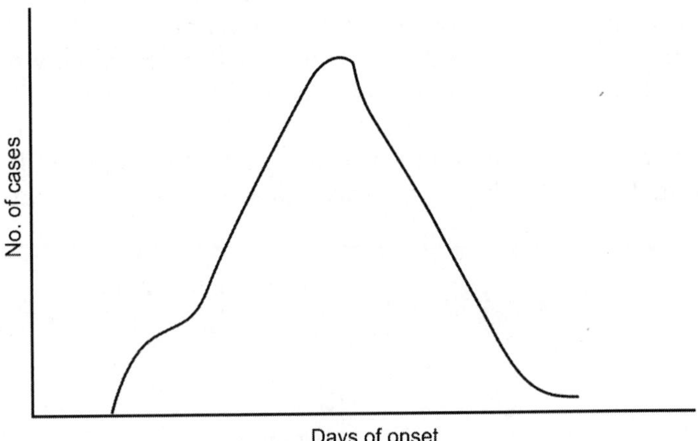

Fig. 2.3: Point source epidemic curve

approximately one-forth of the median incubation period for that disease. The types of epidemic curves are as follows:

- *Point source* (Figs 2.2 and 2.3): In this, there is a close clustering of cases. Example is that of food poisoning cases. The epidemic curve has a sharp upslope, a well-defined peak and a trailing down slope. The peak coincides with the median incubation period. The time of exposure may be bracketed by:

- Counting back the median incubation period from the peak.
- Minimum incubation period from the initial cases.
- Maximum incubation from the last case.

If a point source outbreak of communicable diseases produces a number of infected individuals they may act as sources of infection to others. Secondary cases will appear as a prominent wave separated from the point source peak by approximately a time of one incubation period.

- *Common continuous source* (Figs 2.4 and 2.5): In such cases infection transmits from common sources that continue overtime such as infection of persons from infected food handler. In epidemic curve of such cases rise may be graded or sharp and the peak is generally a gradual plateau. The downslope may be sudden and sharp if the common source is removed or may be a gradual downslope if the source becomes not infective over a period of time.

Propagated (Figs 2.6 and 2.7): This is noticed in cases where disease agents are communicable between persons either directly or through an intermediate vehicle. The cases may be small to start with and increase gradually (depicted by a gradual curve). The curve encompasses several incubation

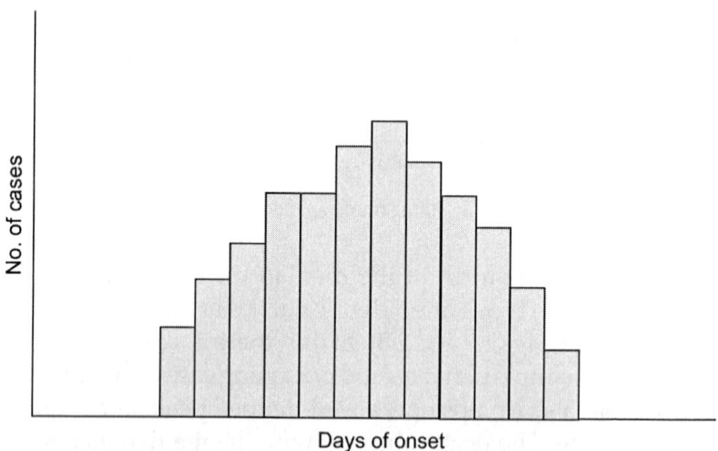

Fig. 2.4: Common source continuous histogram

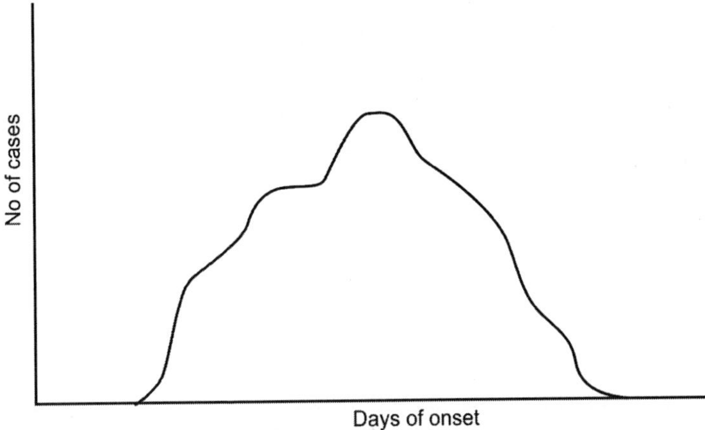

Fig. 2.5: Common source continuous epidemic curve

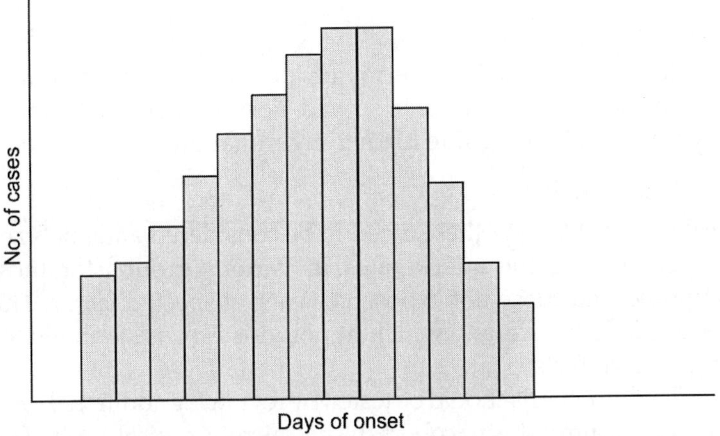

Fig. 2.6: Propagated histogram

periods. After the peak, exhaustion of infective sources usually results in a rapid down slope.

Formulation of Hypothesis

On the basis of time, place and person distribution or the Agent-Host-Environment model, hypothesis should be formulated to

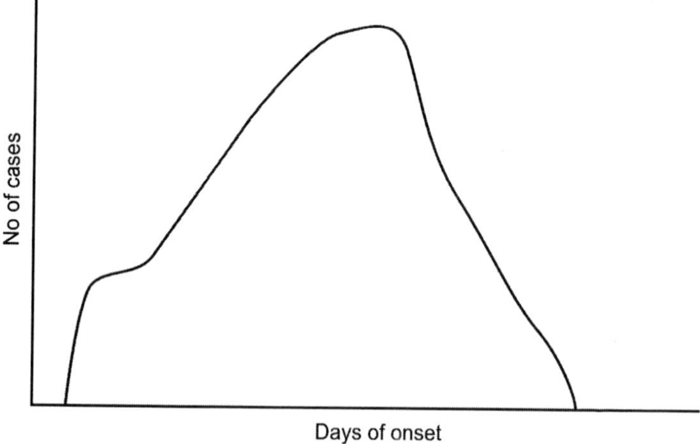

Fig. 2.7: Propagated epidemic curve

explain the epidemic in terms of, possible source, causative agent and possible modes of spread. Formulation of a tentative hypothesis should guide further investigation.

Testing of Hypothesis

All reasonable hypothesis need to be considered and analyzed by comparing the attack rates in various groups for those exposed and those not exposed to each suspected factor. This will enable to ascertain which hypothesis is consistent with all the known facts.

The hypothesis should be tested by reviewing additional cases in a case control study/cohort study/microbiological study. This includes identifying a potential exposure (type and route) for the outbreak and testing this hypothesis using statistical methods. A case control study is the most common approach to hypothesis testing. This compares the frequency of a risk factor in a group of cases (individuals with the nosocomial infection) and in a group of controls (individuals without the infection). The strength of association between exposure and disease is quantified by the odds ratio in case control studies (or the relative risk for cohort studies) with a 95 percent confidence interval. The role of chance, confounding and bias should be considered in interpreting results. Additional data from these studies should be analysed and the hypothesis confirmed or altered.

Evaluation of Ecological Factors

Ecological factors which have made the epidemic possible should be investigated. A detailed environment assessment of the area is also made, e.g. in investigating an epidemic due to cholera, assessment is also made of community water supply system, disposal system, hygienic conditions of cook houses, restaurants, etc.

Further Investigations

A study of the population at risk or a sample of it may be needed to obtain additional information. This may involve medical examination, screening tests, examination of suspected food, faeces/blood samples, biochemical studies, and assessment of immunity status, etc. The approach may be retrospective or prospective.

Control and Prevention

It is essential that steps are taken for immediate control of the outbreak. Measures for prevention should also be enunciated. These should be undertaken concurrently with other measures of managing an outbreak. The main considerations in control and prevention are:

- *Source of infection:* It should be identified at the earliest. Detection and treatment of cases, carrier isolation (if required), and appropriate notification are actions recommended. Control and elimination of source such as food articles, zoonotic reservoir should also be considered. The relevant actions for controlling transmission of the disease should be taken such as checking water supply, food hygiene, appropriate disposal of waste (solid, biomedical, excreta), disinfections/sterilization procedures.
- *Susceptible population:* Appropriate protective measures such as personal protective measures, immunization, immunoprophylaxis, and chemoprophylaxis should be initiated.

Box 2.2: Suggestive format of writing a report

- Information regarding time, geographical area, demographic and health status of the community prior to the outbreak.
- Details of the members of the investigation team.
- Data of number of cases, sex, age, demographic profiling, specimen collection and laboratory testing.
- Attack rate, fatality rate.
- Important observations and findings.
- Specific measures and strategic adopted to control the outbreak.
- Immediate follow-up actions including rehabilitation measures if required.
- Measures and strategies to prevent future outbreaks.
- Conclusion.

- *Preventive strategy:* Surveillance system should be developed and implemented.
- *Information:* On termination of the outbreak information should be given to all concerned.
- *Writing the report:* A detailed report should be written and submitted to appropriate authorities. This should include the background, historical data, methodology of investigations, analysis of data, control measures and recommendations. A suggested format for writing a report after a disease outbreak is shown in Box 2.2.

HOSPITAL INFECTION CONTROL TEAM

It is a team of trained personnel specialized in infection prevention and control of healthcare associated infections. It has following roles.

- Developing, implementing policies, procedures and guidelines on infection prevention and control, and hospital outbreak plans.
- Educating and training of hospital staff on infection prevention and control.
- Surveillance of healthcare associated infection.

When an outbreak is suspected the infection control team (ICT) should conduct as assessment. If outbreak is unlikely,

Box 2.3: Terms of reference–HOCT

- To review evidence and confirm if there is an outbreak based on the case definition established.
- To develop a strategy to deal with the outbreak and to allocate individual responsibilities for implementing actions.
- To investigate the outbreak and identify the nature, vehicle and source of infection.
- To decide control measures including appropriate isolation of patients/ contracts and closure of premises and to monitor their effectiveness in dealing with the cause of the outbreak and in preventing further spread. Practicality, sustainability and service implications should be considered when the infection control measures are recommended.
- To give support and advice on nursing and medical care of patients and to provide specific for patients attendants, visitors, staff and hospital departments where apropriate.
- To ensure adequate staff and resources are available for the management of the outbreak.
- To consider the potential staff training opportunities of the outbreak.
- To identify and utilize any opportunities for the acquisition of new knowledge about disease control.
- To provide support, advice and guidelines to all individuals and organizations directly involved in dealing with the outbreak, which may include general community, hospital patients, visitors, relatives and staff.
- To keep relevant outside agencies, the general public and the media appropriately informed.
- To declare the conclusion of the outbreak and to prepare a final report.
- To evaluate the response to the outbreak and implement changes in OCT procedures based upon lessons learnt.

surveillance should be continued. If an outbreak is noted the hospital outbreak control plan should be activated and hospital outbreak control team (HOCT) convened. Terms of reference of HOCT are enumerated in Box 2.3.

OUTBREAK CONTROL TEAM

Hospitals may need to set-up an outbreak control team (OCT) for both intramural as well as extramural activities. The team serves as a coordinative focal point for health initiatives

Box 2.4: Role of outbreak control team (OCT)

- Deciding whether there is really an outbreak.
- Deciding on the type of investigations to be conducted.
- Case finding and interviews.
- Planning the appropriate clinical and environmental sampling.
- Identifying population at risk and persons likely to act as a source of spreading the infection.
- Ensuring that collaborators use complementary methodology.
- Conducting an environmental investigation of suspected food premises.
- Implementing control measures to prevent further spread by means of exclusions, withdrawal of foods, closure of premises, etc.
- Working in concert with local medical providers to make recommendations on treatment and/or prophylaxis.
- Organizing ongoing communications among OCT members about the outbreak.
- Making arrangements for liaison with the media.
- Producing reports, including lessons learned.
- Requesting external assistance, e.g. secondment of a national.

related to safeguarding the public through sensitization about the problem, symptoms and early diagnosis. The healthcare institutions work alongside the government health agencies and monitoring cells.

Exchange of data and planning are two chief activities of OCT. In the planning process, it is to be ascertained the role that OCT would be playing in collaboration with the disaster management team/ICT, which many institutions may already have. As a disaster may lead to a disease outbreak, it is always beneficial to determine what would be the strategy deployed by the OCT when working with the disaster management team/ICT as well as while working independently.

An important facet of the work of the outbreak control team in a hospital is to organize rapid and systematic treatment of the affected patients who form the influx of the outbreak. Outbreaks may demand extension of services and reorganization of the existing facilities.

The role of the OCT is to coordinate all the activities involved in the investigation and control of an outbreak. This may involve the tasks listed in Box 2.4.

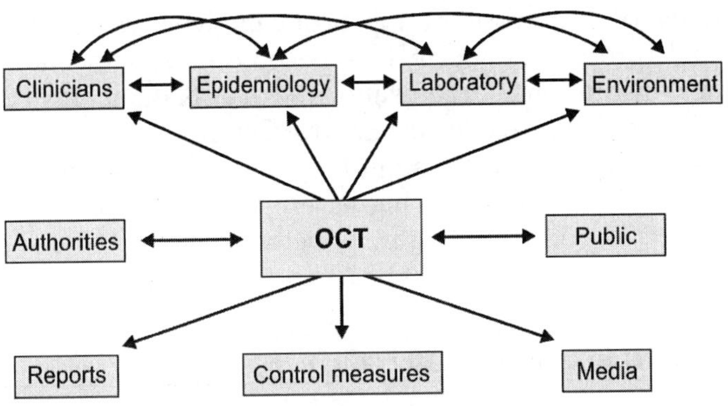

Fig. 2.8: Coordinating role of the OCT

The coordination role of the OCT in an outbreak investigation has been shown in Figure 2.8.

The health authority in the area that first identified and reported the outbreak may initiate the establishment of an OCT. In an outbreak that crosses administrative boundaries, the team should determine at its first meeting, who is represented on the team and should identify the individual who will act as chairperson. Once established, the OCT should be in charge of all investigation and control activities. Members constituting OCT will vary according to circumstances but should normally include a public health practitioner or epidemiologist, a specialist in laboratory medicine (microbiologist, toxicologist, or others as appropriate), a hospital administrator and a senior member of the nursing services. In addition, one or more of the following may be needed according to the nature of the outbreak:

- Food scientist (chemist, food microbiologist, technologist), clinician, veterinarian, toxicologist, virologist, other technical experts, public relations officer, representatives of local authorities, hospital director, and members of hospital infection control team.

OCT also gathers data of incidence to determine whether the incidence threshold is within the limits of disease outbreak definition. However, preparation, detection, response and evaluation remain the core strategies for an operational OCT at primary, secondary as well as tertiary levels of healthcare delivery. With appropriate approvals, and when required OCT through proper channel needs to coordinate with National bodies/Institutions/Organizations such as National Institutes of Virology, National Poison Control Centre.

Depending on the magnitude of the disease outbreak, OCT may be formed at a higher authoritative level such as a district. The decision hierarchy between District, Block and Institution level OCTs must be clearly specified.

IMPORTANT PROCESSES AND FACILITIES

After defining the scope of the disease and taking the initial steps, a few important components/processes/infrastructure needs to be included in the hospital outbreak management plan.

Coordination

Very often, due to the workload and due to lack of an early understanding of the disease, prevalence and manifestation, there is a potential chance of the early cases, which contribute maximum to the spread, remaining undiagnosed or misdiagnosed. Hence, a hospital administrator should develop good coordination with the laboratory (internal or outsourced) so that pathologic correlation could be ascertained.

Categorization

The staff and patients may be grouped into three groups viz. "Ill", "Exposed" (not ill, but in incubation period) and "Not ill/not exposed". The healthcare facility should not admit new patients if there are no facilities to segregate "not ill/not exposed" and "ill/exposed" exhorts. Community dining or recreational activities should also be suspended.

Promptness in Diagnostic Investigations

There should be promptness of the delivery of the investigation results. If the results are delayed to an extent that the patient leaves the hospital, it would not only be waste of laboratory resources but will also be a potential source of unidentified contamination through the patient. However, in such circumstances, taking detailed demographic history from the patient will help the hospital in providing (if required) the health authorities, the information which could be one major step in preventing the disease from spreading. Periodic updates from the laboratory should be received both by the treating physicians as well as the administrative authorities. In case, laboratory testing demands for highly expensive/ elaborate tests, immediate efforts must be made to procure the reagents/kits/chemicals. Assistance in procurement from state/central/municipal/district government authorities should also be explored.

Special Facilities

If the patient is admitted in a hospital, depending upon the laboratory diagnosis and other clinical investigations, immediate action needs to be taken to transfer the patient to the isolation ward. Isolation is an activity instituted to prevent the spread of infection from the patient to other patients. This calls for negative pressure in the isolation ward. The concept of reverse isolation is to ensure that the patient, who could be acutely or chronically immune deficient, does not get infections from other sources including healthcare workers. This arises the need for a positive pressure isolation wards. Depending upon the health and immune status of the patient, a suitable choice should be made by the hospital administrator. Once the patients have been isolated, barrier nursing must be instituted and adequate arrangements need to be taken to prevent and contact between the patient and visitors/healthcare workers, who are not involved in the patient management process.

Screening of Staff

Efforts must be made by the management to screen the health of those workers who are selected to manage an isolation ward in an outbreak situation. This would include their medical history, infection status, immunization status and nutritional status. Staff with sign/symptoms suggestive of being infected by the disease should not be allowed to take part in patient care activities.

Epidemiological Linkage

Environment and local conditions will play a vital role is both problem definition as well as in solution implementation. It would be an inevitable step for the health/hospital administrators to correlate the finding of the cases with the source. For it is the identification and thereby isolation of the unknown/known source that would lead to an effective control of the disease. Advice should be taken from epidemiologists to understand/analyze the disease cycle and implement an effective policy.

Communication

Effective communication is an essential facet. Timely and appropriate communication allay panic amongst the public, prevent spread of rumours, confusion, and also reduces morbidity and mortality. On a global perspective effective communication minimizes the adverse publicity and encourages support.

Equipment

Equipment and supplies including linen and cleaning material such as mops should be restricted to their specific areas. Use of items such as blood pressure cuffs should be for individual patients or disinfected prior to use on another patient.

Activity Flow Charts

The performance of a healthcare institution is greatly influenced if a schedule of activity is planned and corresponding flow chart of these activities is communicated to the various providers of healthcare. Thus, preparing a chart for outbreak management plan, decision matrix or activity flow charts would be greatly useful. The main stages that need to be considered are depicted in Figure 2.9.

EPIDEMIC FORECASTING

Forecasting of an epidemic is done by various methods including sophisticated statistical and operational research

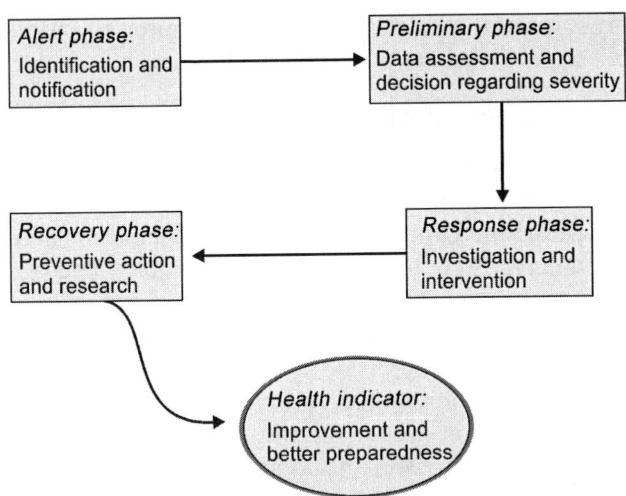

Fig. 2.9: Phases of a disease outbreak

techniques. Such methods and techniques are beyond the purview of this book. Early forecasting of an epidemic is possible by methodical surveillance. Prompt intervention on the basis of the surveillance reports may even abort or at least contain the epidemic before it reaches its peak. Surveillance is of paramount importance in epidemic forecasting and its management.

Definition

Surveillance is continued watchfulness over the distribution and trends of the incidence, by systematic collection, consolidation and evaluation of health data, as well as regular dissemination of interpretations to all concerned. It utilizes methods which have practicability, uniformity and rapidity, rather than complete accuracy. The term "surveillance and monitoring" are often used interchangeably but they are, in fact, distinct. Monitoring refers to ongoing measurements of health services or health program with a view to 'evaluate' the particular program/service or intervention, with constant adjustment of performance in relation to the result. In addition, surveillance concerns general populations while monitoring applies to specific target groups (e.g. vaccinated infants).

Techniques of Forecasting

The techniques of forecasting of epidemic are based on the trend analysis of the particular disease over a period of time. Sophisticated forecasting methods including based on operational research techniques are available. These, being outside the scope of this book are not described. Simple operational measures which may be undertaken for forecasting are:

- Tabulation of the data on monthly basis and yearly basis for at least three years on the following parameters of immediate comparison and identifying the deviations:
  - Disease.
  - Sex.
  - Age group.
  - Incidence/prevalence rate of the disease for the same months of the past three years.
  - Regional, State and National incidence/prevalence rates/ratios of relevant diseases during past years.
- Comparison of monthly and year wise data based on available rates/ratios.
- Plotting different graphs for total, sex-wise, age group-wise incidence and prevalence for the past few years.
- Preparing spot maps to detect regional variation, if any.
- Comparing seasonal and cyclic variations with respect to specific disease.

EPIDEMIC INTELLIGENCE

Epidemic intelligence provides a conceptual framework within which countries may adapt their public health surveillance sytem to meet new challenges. This approach represents a new paradigm aiming at complementing the traditional surveillance systems. Epidemic intelligence (EI) encompasses all activities related to early identification of potential health hazards, their verification, assessment and investigation in order to recommend public health control measures. EI integrates both an indicator-based as well as an event-based component. 'Indicator-based component' refers to structured data collected through routine surveillance systems, whereas 'event-based component' refers to unstructured data gathered from sources of intelligence of any nature. The first step is data collection (indicator-based component) and the detection/capture of events (event-based component). Data collection refers to quantitative indicators (number of cases, rates, etc.) routinely obtained from established surveillance systems. It may also include qualitative research methods like focused group discussions.

CHAPTER

Responsibilities of Hospital Administrators

Hospitals continue to be the first line of responders in any disease outbreak and the response of the hospital is greatly influenced by the hospital administrators and healthcare policy decision-makers. The response needs to be based on scientific, evidence-based and accepted norms. Hospital administrators have a vital role in managing disease outbreaks. The responsibilities and duties are multifaceted. Some of the components which need focus are enumerated below.

TEAM WORK

The hospital administrator should utilize the Outbreak Control Team (OCT) for initiating effective response. OCT would have the most complete information of events and disease episodes, thus making it the appropriate team to communicate all aspects of the disease profile and therapeutic measures taken, to the concerned public health authorities. The official spokesperson of the hospital/healthcare facility should be a member of the OCT. The OCT may have one or more Quick Reaction Teams (QRTs). QRTs are given authority to initiate action under a preset protocol, to minimize death, disability and/or infection. Emergency medical response preparedness includes plan for initial patient evaluation and admission, isolation and treatment modalities. Through appropriate channel, it may be desirable for the OCT to coordinate with higher authorities such as the Ministry of Health and Family Welfare and Directorate General, Health Services, to ensure that the micro plan for response is in consonance with the guidelines issued by the National Authorities.

SPECIAL FACILITIES

A suitable location, separate from other clinical triage and evaluation areas should be identified for the triage of patients that are suspected to be a victim of disease outbreak. If CBRN (Chemical, Biological, Radiological and Nuclear) outbreaks are suspected, it would be desirable to ensure use of decontamination chambers before entering this triage facility. Coordination with the National Disaster Management Authority (NDMA) and adherence to protocols issued by NDMA is also recommended to ensure safety of patients as well as that of health workforce.

STANDARDIZATION

Issuance of latest available clinical guidelines pertaining to case definitions, treatment protocols and prophylaxis, will initiate/ augment awareness among the healthcare professionals.

LABORATORY SERVICES

Laboratory requirement should be as per the diagnostic needs. In case tests specific to disease confirmation are not available, arrangement should be made to collaborate with an accredited laboratory to ensure prompt and evidence-based management. Laboratory sample collection unit needs adequate monitoring. Standard Operating Protocols (SOPs) should be available and implemented for action. Identification and stocking of likely medicines/vaccines and other laboratory assay requirements, RT-PCR, virus isolation, and immuno-fluorescence antibody assays, etc. is required to keep the diagnostic and therapeutic facilities fully operational. However, this could be done after assessing the demand of the cases in a healthcare facility and needs to be in consonance with the level of care that is being provided in the facility.

INVENTORY MANAGEMENT

A disease outbreak may escalate the market price of medical items, e.g. during H_1N_1 outbreak there was a significant increase in the price of facemasks. There were some hospitals that had to cancel planned surgeries due to shortage of masks. The demand of disease specific items become highly elastic, i.e.

a small increase in the demand greatly increases the price per unit, as the supply does not increase proportionately. It would be advisable to estimate the demand and supply position and stock the items accordingly. Forecast of any future need (incase the episode prolongs), should be made on the basis of usage reports collected from various consumption centers of the healthcare facility. Batch number of the items used during the period of outbreak needs to be especially monitored for the quality and consistency in quality. Any complaints regarding the same should be immediately reported as a lapse in any of the quality dimensions of the product will have an impact on a large patient community. Stores having rate contracts with suppliers for inventory maintenance of drugs will be helpful in keeping the budget predictable. The hospital administrator needs to take stock of the essential drugs and medications. It would be helpful for the hospital to keep appropriate buffer stock of medications at least those that are prescribed in the "National list of essential drugs" and/or "WHO list of essential drugs". Logistics and supply chain might get affected during the period of disease outbreak. Similarly, if the treatment necessitates use of life-saving equipment like ventilators, etc. the need has to be ascertained. It is not always possible to have all expensive equipment as buffer stock, on a fulltime basis in large numbers, to be used for a short time period as in a disease outbreak situation. During such circumstances, taking the equipment on rental contract basis could be an alternative option. This could be done from the manufacturers or from other hospitals which have the equipment in sufficient or surplus number. Incase a hospital has adequate equipment, it is necessary to maintain them functional and undertake preventive maintenance.

SECURITY OF STORES

Security of stores needs to be upgraded during the disease outbreak. During the period of high consumption, and increased footfalls there are likely to be more chances of potential thefts and pilferage. Security personnel should be appropriately briefed to facilitate effectiveness in security measures.

BUDGET

An additional budgetary allocation may be required by the healthcare facility to cater to the upsurge in patient load.

STAFF HEALTH SAFETY

Health of the hospital staff is of significant importance. Healthcare workers have very high chance of contracting the disease which is prevalent in the community as an outbreak. Healthcare workers falling ill not only add to the patient load and disease burden but also negatively impacts the health workforce needed to restrict and combat the disease. Adequate instructions should be provided to the staff for self-protection from infectious agents. Personal protective materials like masks, gowns, vaccines should be earmarked for the staff of the healthcare facility. The health administrator needs to be extra cautious regarding the health of pregnant female staff. Attention is required towards periodic health screening of the staff through clinical and/or diagnostic means. Education and immunization of staff ensures a healthy and effective human resource in the hospital.

STERILIZATION PROCEDURES

Sterilization procedures should be rechecked for conformance of all prescribed standards. Recall policy for all critical items in case of any lapse in sterilization procedure should be reinforced. In healthcare facilities where test of sterilization is done using biological markers on a weekly basis, the frequency of testing could be increased for the period of high prevalence of the disease. Regular disinfection of semi-critical items and thorough cleaning of noncritical items needs to be done at fixed intervals and a report of preventive and corrective actions should be submitted to the administration.

BLOOD BANK

Strengthening of blood bank of the hospitals remains one of the imperatives of prime importance during the outbreak episode, e.g. during an outbreak of dengue fever, the requirement of platelets goes up in hospitals; hence a sufficient supply of blood through voluntary blood donors ensures meeting the demands of blood and blood components. However, in times of an outbreak, donor screening and blood testing criteria need to be strictly adhered to, so that transfused blood or blood components do not become a medium of spread of the infection.

NETWORKING

Networking greatly facilitates handling capacity of the healthcare institutions during the outbreak. Some of the functions that help effective networking of hospitals and healthcare facilities include complete data collection regarding disease profile and patient demographic details; prompt first aid and structured referral; rehabilitative measures and planning for the safety of the affected patients after their discharge from the hospital(s).

BIOMEDICAL WASTE MANAGEMENT

Scientific disposal of hospital waste is an area requiring alertness. Waste should be handled as per the Biomedical Waste Management Rules prescribed by the Government of India. Segregation at the point of generation, disinfection and categorization is recommended.

REPORTING

Clinical and statistical reporting is a great aid in ascertaining the current status of disease. It provides vital inputs which aids resource pooling and policy framework. Reporting of incidence, treatment given, number of patients refused treatment/admission, and resource adequacy become inputs for facility planning and resource estimation. Accuracy in reports leads to perfection in planning. Reporting needs to be as close to reality as possible, to give an accurate picture of the scenario. The reports need to be authorized by an administrative head. Before forwarding these reports for further action it is to be ensured that the reports have been subjected to a thorough check to eliminate any chance of error. It is for this reason that a hospital administrator must choose a very responsible person to gather the data and make reports. While making the report, it should be ensured that past occurrences of similar or different outbreaks do not cast any influences thus tainting the results with a bias of assumption. Medical records of the patients should be preserved until clearance of disposal is obtained from a competent authority. These records form sources of research studies focused on preventive medicine and epidemiology. Reporting of notifiable disease should be continued through proper channel during the outbreaks. A desirable aspect regarding notifiable diseases reporting is that the forms used by municipal hospitals, state-run hospitals, central government hospitals and autonomous institutions as well as private hospitals need to be standardized. The standardization should be based on national health profile, emerging diseases, rare diseases as well as neglected diseases.

MEDIA MANAGEMENT

There should be a spokesperson to represent a healthcare facility or a hospital. It is advisable that the hospital administrator should follow-up all the media reports and be ready with an authentic and transparent version of the scenario. It is the mismanagement and tampering of the correct report which leads to wrong predictions and panic triggering forecasts. Thus it is important that the reports have brevity, clarity and accuracy. This will eliminate much of the associated ambiguity. However, all information should not be disclosed to general public without the permission of government and/or public health authority. Information that may be true but would certainly lead to panic among patients and vulnerable sections of the society must be kept confidential and be subjected to an assessment of the pros and cons of its disclosure. Such information should be given to the public after necessary permission from the concerned authority. Ideally, all

Box 3.1: Essentials for media management

- Understand the needs of media, notably deadlines and specific requirements of print media, radio, television, and web/internet.
- Coordinate information between agencies involved in the outbreak.
- Appoint a single spokesperson.
- Identify what the main message(s) are for the communication. This message is the single overriding communication objective (SOCO). It must be ensured that the SOCO is clearly stated, in simple language and in a brief well-defined sentence to make it easy for the journalist or editor to insert into news bulletins.
- Be proactive, e.g. by announcing findings with a press release or calling a press conference.
- Manage a regular flow of information updates, e.g. by having a regular briefing time.

such informations should be given to the government health authority and time and extent of its disclosure should be left to its discretion. It is desirable to have a fixed time and date allotted for the media briefing to avoid speculations and related effects. The briefing given to media should be posted on the official website of the healthcare facility to ensure transparency and eliminate distortions/miscommunication. General strategies to improve media communication are listed in Box 3.1.

AMBULANCE SERVICES

Ambulance availability status needs to be evaluated. In case, the healthcare facility has adequate ambulances, those that would be engaged in the outbreak relief should be earmarked and standard operating protocol for their functioning should be established. Phone numbers to confirm the availability of the ambulances should be popularized. Apart from meeting the adequacy of items, equipment and medical gases in the ambulance, special precautions should be taken for proper disinfection of the items used for patient transfers during the outbreak. In case a healthcare facility does not have adequate ambulances, efforts should be made for outsourcing, to cater patient referrals and emergencies.

RESEARCH

Data is a set of information that helps in analysis of observation and result in a logical, sequential and rational manner. Of all the types of data, healthcare data has some crucial issues associated with them. Healthcare data need to be handled with extreme care, as patient's profile and disease status is embedded into them. Any leak of healthcare data into unauthorized hands would mean breach of patient privacy. Healthcare data also indicates the trend of a specific disease in an individual as well as its association with population, thus making it a rich source of epidemiological information. Appropriate application of healthcare data may lead to better disease management and care. Using data for immediate patient care seems to be the most practiced method such as using blood/serum value results for deciding medications/ therapy. However, healthcare data application could be considered complete only when it has been used to prevent further incidence or to minimize the incidence of the disease. Therefore, during disease outbreak, it is vital for healthcare organizations to collect, preserve and archive disease associated healthcare data for further research and academic purposes. This data, could be used by authorized healthcare/government agencies to plan for facilities like health-posts, laboratories, healthcare human resource deployment, and also social facilities like isolation camps, drinking water provisioning, sewage systems and disposal mechanisms. Though, it could look time-consuming during the outbreak phase and may be taken as secondary priority due to increased workload, it should be noted that these data would perhaps be the only way to track the disease source and prevent its recurrence.

PRESERVATION OF SAMPLES/SPECIMEN

Specimen should be preserved, to the extent biologically and clinically possible. Their availability could aid in further research related to biological and genomic associations. However, specimen preservation brings to the fact that a specimen remains the source of disease. Thus, the risk associated with its preservation is manifold. These risks could be minimized using a set of well-defined protocols and in a controlled environment. The environmental needs of sample including temperature, pressure, asepsis, light and chemical surrounding is to be determined and stabilized throughout the process of preservation of the specimen. An important aspect is the interaction of specimen with other factors co-existing in the same environment. This could include laboratory reagents, bio-markers, other specimen, equipment and the healthcare workers who work in the area. It is important to not only protect the sample from getting contaminated or lead to contamination but also to maintain a desirable barrier between the specimen and the people working with these specimens. For the specimen collected during disease outbreak, the collection should be planned using inventory earmarked for this purpose. After analysis, disposal needs to be done after neutralizing the sample with a recommended chemical agent and to be disposed through a channel not linked to immediate hospital/public sewage systems. Preservation of the specimen, if done, should be carried out under strict protocols of accessibility to the sample.

OUTREACH CAMPS

These camps could focus on various population-based diagnostics, therapeutics, and education methods. An effort to reach the population using outreach camps, enormously helps in effective management of a disease outbreak.

INITIAL ASSESSMENT

In order to be adequately prepared for a major public health threat, State and local public health agencies need to have several basic capabilities. Public health departments need to have disease surveillance systems and epidemiologists to detect clusters with suspicious symptoms or diseases in order to facilitate early detection of disease and treatment of victims. Laboratories need to have adequate capacity and necessary staff to test clinical and environmental samples in order to identify an agent promptly so that proper treatment can be started and infectious diseases prevented from spreading. All organizations involved in the response must be able to communicate easily with each other as disease events unfold and critical information is acquired, especially in a large-scale infectious disease outbreak. In addition, plans that describe how State and local officials would manage and coordinate an emergency response need to be in place and to have been tested in an exercise, both at the State and local levels as well as at the regional level. Local healthcare organizations, including hospitals, are generally responsible for the initial response to a public health emergency, be it a bioterrorist attack or a naturally occurring infectious disease outbreak. In the event of a large-scale infectious disease outbreak, hospitals and their emergency departments would be on the frontline, and their personnel would take on the role of first responders. Because hospital emergency departments are open 24 hours a day, 7 days a week, exposed individuals are likely to seek treatment from the medical staff on duty. Staff would need to be able to recognize and report any illness patterns or diagnostic clues that might indicate an unusual infectious disease outbreak to their State or local health department. Triage remains one of the key areas of where an outbreak could be restricted. Triage essentially means to prioritize the needs of the patient-based on the severity, promptness of care required and resources available. However, as far as bio-terrorism or disease outbreak connected to a CBRN disaster is concerned, decontamination unit is an absolute necessity. The purpose is to isolate the patients as far as possible from chemical, biological, radiological or nuclear contamination thereby guarding them against severity as well as protecting other patients who may share the same treatment facility as an affected individual.

PHARMACOVIGILANCE

Pharmacovigilance (PV) is defined as the science and activities relating to the detection, assessment, understanding and prevention of adverse effects or any other drug-related problem. The aims of PV are to enhance patient care and patient safety in relation to the use of medicines; and to support public health programmes by providing reliable, balanced information for the effective assessment of the risk-benefit profile of medicines. It calls for spontaneous reporting of ADRs (Adverse Drug Reactions) from patients, clinicians, manufacturers, civil societies, media and any other relevant public bodies. Disease outbreak management plan must include Pharmacovigilance activities which should include ADR reporting, assessment and reaction control mechanism. The importance of detecting and reporting ADRs goes manifold, during a disease outbreak due to the following reasons:

- The quality of drug available in the market could be sub-standard. There is generally a gap between the supply and demand. There is also likelihood of emergence of spurious drugs.
- The inspection procedures might get temporarily relaxed as authorities try to make the required drug available for the patients in the least possible time.
- The over-the-counter sale of drugs increases as more and more people go in for random prophylactic treatment regimes to safeguard their health.

DOCUMENTATION OF OUTBREAKS AND INVESTIGATIONS

Comprehensive documentation of all recognized outbreaks is essential for any disease surveillance system. Reasons for this include:

- National collection of outbreak data facilities recognition of relationships between events occurring in different areas of the country, such as identification of widely dispersed outbreaks.
- Reports can be used to convince health professionals and the public of the need for preventive measures Documentation of outbreaks may be used to evaluate and improve prevention strategies.
- It is rarely, if ever, possible to identify risk factors for diseases from single sporadic cases. Almost all risk factors are identified from investigations of outbreaks or groups of cases.

- Understanding of emerging disease may be improved, especially their modes of transmission and associated risk factors.
- Reports can be used as teaching aids for diseases and outbreak investigation, including identifying how future outbreak investigations may be improved.
- Outbreak investigations are generally improved through the discipline of systematic and comprehensive documentation.
- Local and national statistics on outbreak occurrence can more readily be compiled when a uniform approach to their recording is used.
- It may be necessary for fulfillment of international reporting requirements, especially if the disease is one where eradication is expected.

COORDINATION

Managing disease outbreak requires coordination of various facets including coordination between sectors and jurisdiction, private and public healthcare institutions. In an epidemic surveillance activities may require collaboration between government health workers, private health provides, community leaders, school teachers/police and panchayats. Effective management of disease outbreak requires that directional leadership be provided throughout the event with appropriate coordination, human and technology resource management. The role of Hospital Administrator in Disease Outbreak Management is summarized in Box 3.2.

RECENT TRENDS

Application of Molecular Typing Methods to Trace the Epidemiology of Hospital Infections and in Early Control of Outbreaks

Pathogen typing was done by comparing the phenotypic characteristics of pathogens (e.g., biotypes, serotypes, bacteriophage or bacteriocin types and antimicrobial susceptibility profiles). However, new DNA-based typing techniques are

Box 3.2: Role of hospital administrators: In disease outbreak management

Ensure
- Standardised protocols, SOPs.
- Appropriate reporting to health authorities.
- Adequate supply of pharmaceutical products.
- Appropriate infrastructure for triage and isolation.
- Availability of diagnostic facilities.
- Biomedical waste management.
- Patient and staff safety.
- Utililization of forecasting techniques for prediction of disease outbreaks.
- Scientific surveillance.
- Correct documentation.
- Effective Media Management. Effective communication modes should be utilized and the media should be used constructively.
- Research, and publications.

changing the approach to study nosocomial transmission of microbes. These DNA-based molecular methodologies include Pulsed Field Gel Electrophoresis (PFGE) and other restriction-based methods, plasmid analysis and polymerase chain reaction (PCR)-based typing methods. Establishing clonality of pathogens can aid in the identification of the source of organisms, distinguish infectious from non-infectious strains and distinguish relapse from re-infection. The goal of genotyping is to establish that epidemiologically related isolates collected during an outbreak of nosocomial disease are also genetically related, suggesting that they originated from the same strain. The determination of the unrelated isolates (sporadic infections) avoids triggering unnecessary and costly epidemic investigations.

DESIGNING ISOLATION FACILITIES SPECIFIC FOR INFECTIOUS DISEASES

Special facilities: If the patient is admitted in the hospital, then, depending upon the laboratory diagnosis and other clinical investigations, immediate action needs to be taken to transfer the patient to the isolation ward. This requires a negative pressure in the isolation ward. The concept of reverse isolation is to ensure that the patient, who could be acutely or chronically immune deficient, does not get infections from other sources, patients or healthcare workers. This necessitates positive pressure isolation. Depending upon the disease profile and immune status of the patients, appropriate selection should be made.

Use of appropriate barrier precautions during patient care is to be instituted and restrictions on visitors should be imposed. Environmental/engineering infection control measures like adequate ventilation, proper patient placement (distance between patients >1m), and adequate environmental cleaning augmented with improved hygiene conditions and meticulous monitoring (like culture swabs from wards, procedure rooms) help in preventing spread of the disease within the hospital.

The general ventilation system should be designed and balanced so that air flows from less contaminated to more contaminated areas. The direction of airflow is controlled by creating a lower (negative) pressure in the area into which the flow of air is desired. Negative pressure is attained by exhausting air from an area at a higher rate than air is being supplied. A hospital is a dynamic, not a static, environment and setting an initial offset does not guarantee that negative pressure is always present. Negative pressure in a closed environment can be altered by changing the ventilation system operation or by the opening and closing of the room's doors, corridor doors, or windows. When an operating configuration has been established, it is essential that all doors and windows remain properly closed in the isolation room and other areas (e.g., doors in corridors that affect air pressure) except when persons need to enter or leave the room or area. The only way to guarantee negative pressure is to measure the pressure differential between the isolation room and the corridor. If pressure-sensing devices are used, negative pressure should be verified at least once a month by using smoke tubes or taking pressure measurements (Flow chart 3.1).

Hospital Infection Control team has a special role to play during an outbreak, the hospital infection control team (ICT) should:

- Conduct an assessment of the extent and importance of outbreak.
- Evaluate if there had been significant spread inside the hospital.

Flow chart 3.1: A decision flow chart for air quality assurance

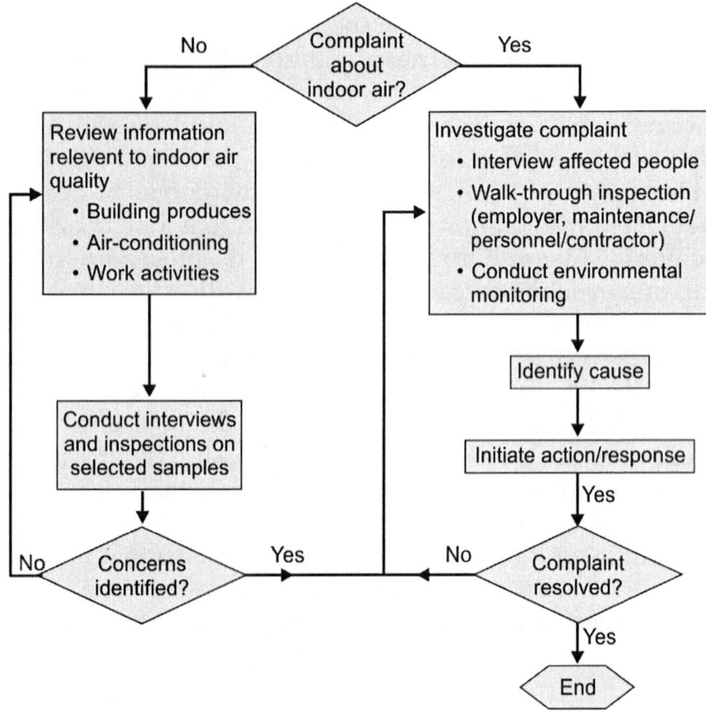

- Ensure that appropriate infection measures are instigated (Personal Protective Equipment (PPE), infection control practices, case finding, contact tracing, surveillance, isolation, cohorting and evaluate their effectiveness in preventing further spread.
- Provide support and advice on nursing and medical care of the patients involved.
- Assess the need for additional resources.

DISEASE OUTBREAKS AND INTERNATIONAL HEALTH REGULATIONS

Notification of Diseases

The primary function of notification is to effect prevention and/or control of the disease. It is a value source of morbidity status. List of notifiable diseases may vary from place to place. Under the International Health Regulations cholera, plague and yellow fever are notifiable to WHO in Geneva. The notifiable diseases as applicable to Greater Mumbai, as per Bombay Municipal Act are listed at Appendix 'A'. The diseases notifiable as per Center for Disease Control (CDC) Atlanta are at Appendix 'B'.

Tuberculosis has recently been made notifiable disease by the Government of India.

Integrated Disease Surveillance Project (IDSP) was launched by Government of India in November 2004. It is a decentralized, State-based Surveillance Program. It is intended to detect early warning signals of impending outbreaks and help initiate an effective response in a timely manner. Major components of the project are:

- Integrating and decentralization of surveillance activities.
- Strengthening of public health laboratories.
- Human Resource Development Training of State Surveillance Officers, District Surveillance Officers, Rapid Response Team, other medical and paramedical staff.
- Use of Information Technology for collection, collation, compilation, analysis and dissemination of data.

For project implementation, Surveillance Units have been set-up at Central, State and District level. Surveillance Committees at National, State and District levels are monitoring the project. Currently linkages are being established with all State Head Quarters, District Head Quarters and all Government Medical Colleges on a Satellite Broadband Hybrid Network. This network enables enhanced Speedy Data Transfer, Video Conferencing, Discussions, Training, Communication and in future e-learning for outbreaks and program monitoring under IDSP. A 24 × 7 call center with toll free telephone no 1075 accessible from BSNL/ MTNL telephone from all States is in operation since February 2008. This receives disease alerts from anywhere in the country and diverges the information to the respective State/District Surveillance Units for verification and initiating appropriate actions wherever required. Under IDSP data is collected on a weekly (Monday—Sunday) basis. The information is collected on three specified reporting formats, namely "S" (suspected cases), "P" (presumptive cases) and "L" (Laboratory confirmed cases) filled by health workers, clinician and clinical laboratory staff. The weekly data gives the time trends. Whenever there is a rising trend of illnesses in any area, it is investigated by the Medical Officers/Rapid Response Teams (RRTs) to diagnose and control the outbreak. Weekly disease surveillance reports are send to Central Surveillance Unit, IDSP. Data analysis and action are being undertaken by respective districts. Emphasis is being laid on reporting of surveillance data from major hospitals both in public and private sectors and also Infectious Disease hospitals. The compilation and disease outbreak alerts are also done.

The International Health Regulations

It is an international legal instrument that is binding on many countries across the globe, including all the Member States of WHO. Their aim is to help the international community prevent and respond to acute public health risks that have the potential to cross borders and threaten people worldwide. The salient features of International Health Regulations (IHR) are as follows:

- In the globalized world, diseases can spread far and wide via international travel and trade. A health crisis in one country can impact livelihoods and economies in many parts of the world. Such crises can result from emerging infections like Severe Acute Respiratory Syndrome (SARS), or a human influenza pandemic. The IHR can also apply to other public health emergencies such as chemical spills, leaks and dumping, or nuclear melt-downs. The IHR aim to limit interference with international traffic and trade while ensuring public health through the prevention of disease spread.
- The IHR, which came into force on 15 June 2007, require countries to report certain disease outbreaks and public health events to WHO. Building on the unique experience of WHO in global disease surveillance, alert and response, the IHR define the rights and obligations of countries to report public health events, and establish a number of procedures that WHO must follow in its work to uphold global public health security.
- The IHR also require countries to strengthen their existing capacities for public health surveillance and response.

WHO is collaborating closely with countries and partners to provide technical guidance and support to mobilize the resources needed to implement the new rules in an effective and timely manner. Timely and open reporting of public health events will help make the world more secure.

- While international travel and trade bring many health benefits linked to economic development, they may also cause public health risks that can spread internationally at airports, ports and ground crossings through persons, baggage, cargo, containers, conveyances, goods and postal parcels.
- The IHR provide a public health response in the form of obligations and standing or temporary nonbinding recommendations in ways that avoid unnecessary interference with international travel and trade.
- IHR recommends strengthen in a public health capacities at designated airports, ports and ground crossings in both routine circumstances and when responding to events that may constitute a public health emergency of international concern.
- It is important for a hospital administrator to know of the IHR so as to enable optimal management of the disease outbreak. In case foreign patients report to Hospitals of India, the Form C (Rule-14) of The Registration of Foreigners Act, 1939 should be duly filled. The copy of this form needs to be sent to the Registration Office of the respective District Headquarters.

Public grievances: Public grievances may increase during an outbreak. This could be because of the scarcity of skilled manpower, overstretching of existing manpower to meet the demand and patient load, constraint of resources, lack of training to meet the outbreak and other related factors. This must be dealt with patience rather than panic. The community's psychological stress often puts the tolerance limit of patients/health workers/resource providers into a lower threshold thus resulting in dissatisfaction. The most effective way is to channelize the faults into methodic grievances which ideally must be made in writing. Thus, many scenarios which are a result of miscommunication could be avoided and the shortcomings as listed in the grievances could be used for strategies of improvement.

CHAPTER

Rating the Preparedness

It is essential that the healthcare institutions are prepared to manage disease outbreaks. It is important to have simple and implementable tools to measure the preparedness of the institution to be able to manage such situations.

CHECKLIST

A checklist has been developed to facilitate the hospital administrations and healthcare providers to rate their preparedness during the disease outbreak. It will also enable them to identify the existing gaps, if any, between the existing and the acceptable/ideal level of preparedness. For evaluation, the following numeric representations are recommended:

Score 0: Cannot be made available/functional/operational.

Score 5: Will be made available/functional/operational within a defined time period.

Score 10: Available/functional/operational.

The maximum/ideal score thus attainable for these checklists is 540. It indicates that the healthcare institution is well-prepared to manage the disease outbreak situation. The score between 450 and 540 indicates that though there are measures in place to generate an outbreak response, however the preparedness status may not be sufficient and further steps need to be taken within a specified time period. The score between 0 and 450 indicates that the healthcare institution needs to undertake systemic measures to be appropriately prepared to manage a disease outbreak. The checklist may be modified to suit evaluation of specific healthcare institutions.

Checklist for Rating the Preparedness

Sl. No.	Components	Rating
1	**Definition and Scope**	
1.1	Is there an existence of concept of Disease Outbreak management (such as availability of disease outbreak management manual)	(10), (5), (0)
2	**Response Initiation**	
2.1	Has Outbreak Control Team been constituted?	(10), (5), (0)
2.2	Has Quick Reaction Team (QRT) been constituted?	(10), (5), (0)
2.3	Are roles assigned to QRTs?	(10), (5), (0)
2.4	Are roles and responsibilities defined for the members of QRT	(10), (5), (0)
3	**Triage**	
3.1	Is there a separate Triage facility?	(10), (5), (0)
3.2	If no Triage area is earmarked, can another area be made ready promptly for triaging?	(10), (5), (0)
3.3	Is there a decontamination unit in Triage facility?	(10), (5), (0)
4	**Prophylaxis and Diagnostic Capability**	
4.1	Are clinical guidelines for treatment protocol and prophylaxis available?	(10), (5), (0)
4.2	Can the confirmatory diagnosis be done in the facility lab?	(10), (5), (0)
4.3	If yes, are reagents/kit adequately available?	(10), (5), (0)
4.4	If no, is there plan for networking/outsourcing?	(10), (5), (0)
4.5	Has the time limit for availability of lab results been specified?	(10), (5), (0)
5	**Medication and Inventory Management**	
5.1	Is there an outbreak disease specific inventory management system?	(10), (5), (0)
5.2	Is there a contingency plan for acute shortage of items?	(10), (5), (0)
5.3	Are life-saving equipment available?	(10), (5), (0)
5.4	If no, any plan for outsourcing?	(10), (5), (0)
6	**Security**	
6.1	Is adequate security deployed in stores?	(10), (5), (0)
6.2	Is adequate security available in patient care areas?	(10), (5), (0)

7	**Networking**	
7.1	Is there networking with other hospitals for exchange of data and resources?	(10), (5), (0)
8	**Finance and Budgeting**	
8.1	Is there a budget provision for additional expenditure due to disease outbreak patient load?	(10), (5), (0)
9	**Indoor Facility**	
9.1	Is there an isolation facility?	(10), (5), (0)
9.2	Has staff been selected and briefed for the isolation area/ward?	(10), (5), (0)
9.3	Is adequate personal protective material available to the staff working in isolation area?	(10), (5), (0)
9.4	Is an area earmarked for in-patients in case of upsurge in disease outbreak patients?	(10), (5), (0)
10	**CSSD (Central Sterile Supply Department)**	
10.1	Is testing of items with biological and/or chemical indicators done and records maintained?	(10), (5), (0)
10.2	Is there a recall policy for defective items after sterilization?	(10), (5), (0)
11	**Blood Bank**	
11.1	Will blood bank be able to provide adequate units of blood/blood components?	(10), (5), (0)
11.2	Is donor screening criteria strict and error free?	(10), (5), (0)
11.3	Is there any networking with other hospitals institutions for blood donation and supply of units of blood and blood components?	(10), (5), (0)
12	**Hospital Waste Management**	
12.1	Is disposal of hospital waste/infectious waste being done as per BMW Rules?	(10), (5), (0)
12.2	Is there staff trained to handle BMW in heavy work load situation?	(10), (5), (0)
13	**Infection Control**	
13.1	Is disinfection of patient utility items done?	(10), (5), (0)
13.2	Are cultures from critical areas being taken?	(10), (5), (0)
13.3	Is there an infection control manual?	(10), (5), (0)
13.4	Is there an infection control team?	(10), (5), (0)
13.5	Is food being supplied to patients subjected to infection check?	(10), (5), (0)

14	**Medical Records and Data Reporting**	
14.1	Is disease reporting format available including form 14 A?	(10), (5), (0)
14.2	Has reporting hierarchy enunciated?	(10), (5), (0)
14.3	Is there a medical records preservation policy?	(10), (5), (0)
14.4	Are International Health Regulation by WHO and IDSP incorporated in the SOP for appropriate reporting?	(10), (5), (0)
15	**Public Relations and Media**	
15.1	Is there a Media Policy?	(10), (5), (0)
16	**Patient Transfer System**	
16.1	Are ambulances earmarked in case of requirement?	(10), (5), (0)
16.2	Does ambulances have necessary equipment?	(10), (5), (0)
16.3	Does SOP exist for checking replenishment/ replacing items?	(10), (5), (0)
17	**Mortuary Arrangement**	
17.1	Is there a facility for keeping dead bodies?	(10), (5), (0)
17.2	Is there a policy for keeping of dead bodies?	(10), (5), (0)
18	**Review**	
18.1	Is there a policy for periodic review of SOPs protocols?	(10), (5), (0)
18.2	Is surveillance of diseases being done?	(10), (5), (0)
19	**Data Management**	
19.1	Is the data received during earlier outbreak, if any, being archived and analyzed for further research?	(10), (5), (0)
19.2	Has documentation of the outbreak been done including any reports, summary, periodic reviews?	(10), (5), (0)
20	**Sample/ specimen storage**	
20.1	Are samples/specimen storage SOPs/protocols available?	(10), (5), (0)
21	**Outreach Camps**	
21.1	Has outreach camps been planned for diagnosis, treatment, health education and/or surveillance?	(10), (5), (0)
22	**Pharmacovigilance**	
22.1	Is there a system for reporting adverse drug reactions?	(10), (5), (0)

CONCLUSION

The number of outbreaks and their extent can impact healthcare systems. Disease outbreaks often cause public health emergencies with resultant increased morbidity and mortality. Disease outbreaks cannot always be predicted or prevented, however, timely investigations and specific measures may limit the spread and adverse effects of the outbreak.

It is certain that in future diseases would spread rapidly between Continents, Countries, States and Districts facilitated by the modern day air travel and other modalities of transport. There would be simultaneous impact on all communities. High population density would further augment it. The high strike rate would generally overwhelm the resource of healthcare facilities. Limited availability of drugs and vaccines would accentuate the crisis situation. Sickness absenteeism or otherwise would have impact on all sectors. Socio-economic disruption would ensue. Hospital administrators must ensure that the hospital or the healthcare facility provides prompt and correct treatment to the patients affected by a disease outbreak. Appropriate preparedness of the healthcare facility as well as that of the community will facilitate in managing disease outbreaks effectively. A directional leadership along with operational and strategic preparedness will enable hospital administrators to prevent/mitigate/control disease outbreaks.

Glossary

Antimicrobial resistance rate: For multiple-drug-resistant bacteria surveillance, the three main indicators used are percentage of antimicrobial-resistant strains within isolates of a species, for example, percentage of MRSA, attack rate (e.g. Number of BSI/100 admissions) and incidence rate (e.g. BSI/1000 patient-days).

For both prevalence and incidence rates, either the entire population under surveillance or only patients with a specific risk exposure may be the denominator. Incidence rates include the length of exposure or the length of stay (and/or follow-up) of the patient. They give a better reflection of risk and facilities comparisons.

Attack rate (cumulative incidence rate): This is defined as the number of new infections acquired in a period/number of patients observed in the same period × 100.

Cluster: Aggregation of relatively uncommon events or disease in space and/or time in amounts that are believed or perceived to be greater than could be expected by chance.

Cohort: Group of individuals sharing a common characteristic.

Epidemic curve: This is constructed to study the epidemic pattern of the disease. An epidemic curve is a graph in which the cases of disease that occurred during the outbreak are plotted according to time of onset of the cases. The epidemic curve is constructed to help determine whether the source of infection is common and continuing and identify the probable time of exposure of the cases to the source of infection and probable incubation period.

Epidemic study-cohort study: Depending upon the infection problem, a defined high-risk population (cohort) is identified and followed prospectively. This high-risk population is followed prospectively for the development of infection. After following these cases for some time, the differences in host factors between the patients that develop the infection and those that do not becomes evident and will identify the source of the problem.

Epidemic study-case control study: A group of uninfected patients (the control group) is compared with infected patients (the case group). The differences in characteristics, susceptibility and exposure factors are compared. These factors include age, sex, time, place, duration of stay, intervention, antibiotic therapy and other therapies. A statistically significant difference between the groups is identified and the problem can be delineated.

Epidemiology: Study of the frequency, distribution and determination of disease and health problems in human population and its application in prevention, control and mitigation of health problems.

Healthcare-associated infection: Infection that patients may have acquired during the course of receiving treatment for other conditions within a healthcare setting (formerly referred to nosocomial infections).

Incidence rates: This is defined as the number of new nosocomial infections acquired in a period/total number of patient-days for the same period × 1000 (e.g. Incidence of VAP for 1000 ventilator-days or incidence of MRSA for 10,000 patient-days).

Monitoring: Term 'surveillance' and 'monitoring' are often used interchangeably but they are, in fact, distinct. Monitoring refers to ongoing measurements of health services or a health programme with a view to 'evaluate' the particular programme/service or interventions, with constant adjustment of performance in relation to the results. In addition, surveillance concerns general populations while monitoring applies to specific target groups (e.g. vaccinated infants).

Outbreak: The perceived or true occurrence of more cases of a communicable disease than expected in a given area or among a specific group of people over a defined period of time.

Prevalence rates: This is defined as the number of infected patients (or number of infections) at the time of study/number of patients observed at the same time x 100 (e.g. Prevalence [%] of HAI for 100 hospitalized patients).

Reservoir: The reservoir is 'any person, animal arthropod, plant, soil, any environment site or substance, or a combination of these, in which an infectious agent normally lives and multiples; on which it depends primarily for survival; and from which it could be transferred directly or indirectly to a susceptible host. It is the natural habitat of the infectious agent'. Reservoirs do not necessarily transmit infection, unless they are a potential source. Removal or destruction of a reservoir does not prevent transmission of infection, unless it is also a potential source. It is generally accepted that the source is the part of reservoir.

Spot map: A map represented by dots where each dot represents a case or some other incident of epidemiological interest. Map of the areas where possibly the exposure of disease could have happened is made. Frequency of the disease is plotted as dots. Actual number of cases may also be plotted rather than the frequency.

Source: The source of infection is defined as 'the person, animal, object, site or substance, where a pathogen may grow and from which they are transmitted to colonize or cause an infection at another site of the same person or in another person'. Sources are usually infected or colonized patients or staff, or less frequently, the inanimate environment (infected wounds, the nose or faces of a carrier, contaminated food, contaminated water, etc.). Identification of the correct source is essential to arrest the spread from this source.

Standard precautions: Standard precautions are work practice implemented to achieve a basic standard of infection control to minimize the transmission of infections in healthcare institution. They can reduce the potential for transmission of infection from person to person, whether patients, nursing, medical/allied health or other staff members. These practices are to be used during the care of all patients in all healthcare settings, regardless of the suspected or confirmed presence of an infectious agent. These are based on the principle that all blood, body fluids, secretions, excretions except sweat, non-intact skin and mucous membranes may contain transmissible infectious agents. Although initially developed for the protection of healthcare personnel, the new elements of standard precautions focus on the protection of patients by ensuring that HCWs do not transfer infectious agents to patients via hands, respiratory tract, blood or equipment during patient care. The elements of standard precautions includes hand hygiene, safe injection practices, worker safety, antimicrobial policy, immunoprophylaxis, biomedical waste management, surveillance of healthcare associated infections.

Surveillance: Continued watchfulness over the distribution and trends of the incident by systematic collection, consolidation and evaluation of health data, as well as regular dissemination of interpretations to all concerned. It is distinguished by methods having practicability, uniformity and rapidity rather than complete accuracy.

Appendices

Appendix 'A'

THE NOTIFIABLE DISEASES AS APPLICABLE TO GREATER MUMBAI

1. Small Pox
2. Cholera
3. Plague
4. Enteric fever (Typhoid fever)
5. Scarlet fever
6. Yellow fever
7. Diphtheria
8. Typhus
9. Relapsing fever
10. Puerperal fever
11. Tuberculosis
12. Leprosy
13. Influenza
14. Cerebrospinal fever
15. Poliomyelitis
16. Virus encephalitis
17. Infectious hepatitis
18. Dengue fever
19. Gastroenteritis
20. AIDS
21. Meningococcal meningitis
22. Leptospirosis

Appendix 'B'

THE NOTIFIABLE DISEASES IN 2011 AS PER CDC ATLANTA

1. Anthrax
2. Arboviral neuroinvasive and non-neuroinvasive diseases
   - California serogroup virus disease
   - Eastern equine encephalitis virus disease
   - Powassan virus disease
   - St. Louis encephalitis virus disease
   - West Nile virus disease
   - Western equine encephalitis virus disease
3. Babesiosis
4. Botulism
   - Botulism, foodborne
   - Botulism, infant
   - Botulism, other (wound and unspecified)
5. Brucellosis
6. Chancroid
7. *Chlamydia trachomatis infection*
8. Cholera
9. Coccidioidomycosis
10. Cryptosporidiosis
11. Cyclosporiasis
12. Dengue
    - Dengue fever
    - Dengue hemorrhagic fever
    - Dengue shock syndrome
13. Diphtheria
14. Ehrlichiosis/Anaplasmosis
    - *Ehrlichia chaffeensis*
    - *Ehrlichia ewingii*
    - *Anaplasma phagocytophilum*
    - Undetermined
15. Giardiasis
16. Gonorrhea
17. *Haemophilus influenzae, invasive disease*
18. Hansen disease (leprosy)

19. Hantavirus pulmonary syndrome
20. Hemolytic uremic syndrome, post-diarrheal
21. Hepatitis
    - Hepatitis A, acute
    - Hepatitis B, acute
    - Hepatitis B, chronic
    - Hepatitis B virus, perinatal infection
    - Hepatitis C, acute
    - Hepatitis C, past or present
22. HIV infection*
    - HIV infection, adult/adolescent (age > = 13 years)
    - HIV infection, child (age >= 18 months and < 13 years)
    - HIV infection, pediatric (age < 18 months)
23. Influenza-associated pediatric mortality
24. Legionellosis
25. Listeriosis
26. Lyme disease
27. Malaria
28. Measles
29. Meningococcal disease
30. Mumps
31. Novel influenza A virus infections
32. Pertussis
33. Plague
34. Poliomyelitis, paralytic
35. Poliovirus infection, nonparalytic
36. Psittacosis
37. Q Fever
    - Acute
    - Chronic
38. Rabies
    - Rabies, animal
    - Rabies, human
39. Rubella
40. Rubella, congenital syndrome
41. Salmonellosis
42. Severe Acute Respiratory Syndrome-associated Coronavirus (SARS-CoV) disease

43. Shiga toxin-producing *Escherichia coli (STEC)*
44. Shigellosis
45. Smallpox
46. Spotted Fever Rickettsiosis
47. Streptococcal toxic-shock syndrome
48. *Streptococcus pneumoniae,* invasive disease
49. Syphilis
    - Primary
    - Secondary
    - Latent
    - Early latent
    - Late latent
    - Latent, unknown duration
    - Neurosyphilis
    - Late, non-neurological
    - Stillbirth
    - Congenital
50. Tetanus
51. Toxic-shock syndrome (other than Streptococcal)
52. Trichinellosis (Trichinosis)
53. Tuberculosis
54. Tularemia
55. Typhoid fever
56. Vancomycin-intermediate *Staphylococcus aureus* (VISA)
57. Vancomycin-resistant *Staphylococcus aureus* (VRSA)
58. Varicella (morbidity)
59. Varicella (deaths only)
60. Vibriosis
61. Viral Hemorrhagic Fevers, due to
    - Ebola virus
    - Marburg virus
    - Arenavirus
    - Crimean-Congo Hemorrhagic Fever virus
    - Lassa virus
    - Lujo virus
    - New world arenaviruses (Gunarito, Machupo, Junin, and Sabia viruses)
62. Yellow fever

Appendix 'C'

NATIONAL SURVEILLANCE PROGRAMME FOR COMMUNICABLE DISEASES

The disease burden of the people of India is one of the highest in the world. This is mainly due to the heavy burden of infectious diseases.

Surveillance in Disease Control

- A systematic process of reporting of various diseases of public health importance, as and when, and where, they occur, to a designated agency responsible for taking effective interventional steps, is known as disease surveillance.
- Infectious diseases occur as a result of amplification and transmission of infectious agents. Detecting disease, as, when and where it occurs, and it's clustering, are essential for disease control. Surveillance, in other words, is the first step in intervention. Surveillance is particularly important for the early detection of outbreaks of diseases. In the absence of surveillance, disease may spread unrecognized. By the time the outbreak is recognized, the best opportunity to take intervention measures might have been over.
- Surveillance is essential for the early detection of emerging or reemerging infectious diseases. In the absence of surveillance, individual healthcare workers may not recognize the new disease, but may apply a near-fit diagnosis of a locality prevalent disease, which the disease in question may resemble.

National Institute of Communicable Diseases

National Institute of Communicable Diseases (NICD) had its origin as Central Malaria Bureau, established at Kasauli (Himachal Pradesh) in 1909 and following expansion was renamed in 1927 as the Malaria Survey of India. The organization was shifted to Delhi in 1938 and called as the Malaria Institute of India (MII). In view of the drastic reduction achieved in the incidence of malaria under National Malaria Eradication Programme (NMEP), Government of India decided to reorganize and expand the activities of the Institute to cover other communicable diseases. On 30 July, 1963 the erstwhile MII was renamed as NICD to shoulder these additional responsibilities.

The Institute was established to function as a national center of excellence for control of communicable diseases. The function of the Institute also included various areas of training and research using multidisciplinary integrated approach. The Institute was, in addition, expected to provide expertize to the States and Union Territories (UTs) on rapid health assessment and laboratory-based diagnostic services. Surveillance of communicable diseases and outbreak investigation also formed an indispensable part of its activities.

The Institute is under administrative control of the Director General of Health Services, Ministry of Health and Family Welfare, Govt. of India. The Director, an officer of the Public Health sub-cadre of Central Health Service, is the administrative and technical head of the Institute.

The Institute has its headquarters in Delhi and has 8 out-station branches located at Alwar (Rajasthan), Bengaluru (Karnataka), Kozhikode (Kerala), Coonoor (Tamil Nadu), Jagdalpur (Chhattisgarh), Patna (Bihar), Rajahmundry (Andhra Pradesh) and Varanasi (Uttar Pradesh).

There are several technical divisions at the headquarters of the Institute, i.e. Centre for Epidemiology and Parasitic Diseases (Dept. of Epidemiology, Dept. Parasitic Disease) Division of Microbiology, Division of Zoonosis, Centre for HIV/AIDS and related diseases, Centre for Medical Entomology and Vector Management, Division of Malariology and Coordination, Division of Biochemistry and Biotechnology.

In each division there are several sections and laboratories dealing with different communicable diseases. The divisions have well equipped laboratories with modern equipment capable of undertaking tests using latest technology. The Institute has a 24 × 7 Disease Monitoring Cell operating round the clock to respond to enquiries related to disease outbreak alongwith video-conferencing facility to interact with the network of disease surveillance centers in the states and districts. The branches are also well equipped and staffed to carry out field studies, training activities and research.

The mandate of the Institute broadly covers three areas viz. services, trained health manpower development and research.

Services

The Institute takes leading role in undertaking investigations of disease outbreaks all over the country employing epidemiological and diagnostic tools. It also provides referral diagnostic services to individuals, community, medical colleges, research institutions and state health directorates. The service component provided by the Institute also includes making available scientific research material, teaching aids, storage and supply of vaccines and quality control of biologicals. A brief of different services provided are mentioned below.

Outbreak Investigations

The Institute investigates and recommends control measures for the outbreak of various communicable diseases in the States/UTs all over the country as well as to some neighboring countries in the South East Asia Region. The Institute also undertakes monitoring of outbreaks throughout the country, especially during its early rising phase by collecting information from the states and districts. The Institute conducts emergency preparedness training for the officials in the states as well as investigates rumors in cases of diseases that have been considered as eradicated, e.g. smallpox cases.

Referral Services

Referral Diagnostic Services: The Institute provides referral diagnostic services for various communicable diseases of microbial origin specially for those for which diagnostic facilities are ordinarily not available in hospitals and medical colleges. These include:

Viral diseases: Poliomyelitis, measles, coxsackie virus, other enteroviruses, hepatitis virus, AIDS, rabies, arbo-viral infections, rubella, cytomegalovirus, etc.

Bacterial diseases: Meningitis, diphtheria, acute respiratory infections, cholera and newer enteropathogens, plague, anthrax, brucellosis, rickettsioses, etc.

Mycotic diseases: Common fungal infections, superficial as well as deep.

Parasitic diseases: Malaria, kala-azar, leptospirosis, hydatidosis.

Appendix 'D'

THE EPIDEMIC DISEASES ACT, 1897

ACT NO. 3 OF 1897[1]

[1]{This Act has been amended in its application to –

1. The Punjab by the Epidemic Diseases (Punjab Amendment) Act, 1944 (Punjab Act 3 of 1944); in East Punjab by East Punjab by East Punjab Act 1 of 1947;
2. The CP and Berar by the CP and Berar Epidemic Diseases (Amendment) Act, 1945 (CP and Berar Act 4 of 1945)}

An Act to provide for the better prevention of the spread of Dangerous Epidemic Diseases.

[4th February, 1897]

CONTENTS

Whereas it is expedient to provided for the better prevention of the spread of dangerous epidemic disease; It is hereby enacted as follows:

Short Title and Extent

1. This Act may be called the Epidemic Diseases Act, 1897.

{Subs by the AO 1950} [(2) It extends to the whole of India except *{Subs by the Adaptation of Laws (No 2) Order, 1956 for "Part B States".}* [The territories which, immediately before the 1st November, 1956, were comprised in Part B States.] *{The word "and" at the end of sub-section (2), and sub-section (3), rep by Act 10 of 1914, s3 and SchII}.*

{The word "and" at the end of sub-section (2), and sub-section (3), rep by Act 10 of 1914, s3 and SchII}.

{For notifications issued under this section, see different local Rules and Orders.}

Power to take Special Measures and Prescribe Regulations as to Dangerous Epidemic Diseases

1. When at any time the *{Subs by the AO 1937, for "GG in C"}* [State Government] is satisfied that {Subs, ibid for "India".} [the State] or any part thereof is visited by, or threatened with, an outbreak of any dangerous epidemic disease, the *{Subs by the AO 1937, for "GG in C"}* [State Government, if *{Subs ibid for "he"}* [it] thinks that the ordinary provisions of the law for the time being in force are in sufficient for the purpose, may take, or require or empower any person to take, such measures and, by public notice, prescribe such temporary regulations to be observed by the public or by any person or class of persons as *{Subs ibid for "he"}* [it] shall deem necessary to prevent the outbreak of such disease or the spread thereof, and may determine in what manner and by whom any expenses incurred (including compensation if any) shall be defrayed.
2. In particular and without prejudice to the generality of the foregoing provisions, the *{Subs by the AO 1937, for "GG in C"}* [State Government] may take measures and prescribe regulations for–
   {Paragraph (a) omitted, ibid}
   b. the inspection of persons traveling by railway or otherwise, and the segregation, in hospital, temporary accommodation or otherwise, of persons suspected by the inspecting officer of being infected with any such disease.

{Sub-section (3) omitted by Act 38 of 1920, s2 and SchI}

{Subs by the AO 1937, for s2A ins by Act 38 of 1920, s2 and SchI}.

Power of Central Government

1. When the Central Government is satisfied that Indian or any part thereof is visited by, or threatened with, an outbreak of any dangerous epidemic disease and that the

ordinary provisions of the law for the time being in force are insufficient to prevent the outbreak of such disease or the spread thereof, the Central Government may take measures and prescribe regulations for the inspection of any ship or vessel leaving or arriving at any port in *{Subs by the Adaptation of Laws (No 2) Order, 1956 for "a Part A State or a Part C State"}* [the territories to which this Act extends] and for such detention thereof, or of any person intending to sail therein, or arriving thereby, as may be necessary.

Penalty

Any person disobeying any regulation or order made under this Act shall be deemed to have committed an offence punishable under section 188 of the Indian Penal Code (45 of 1860).

Protection to Persons Acting Under Act

No suit or other legal proceeding shall lie against any person for anything done or in good faith intended to be done under this Act.

Bibliography

1. Biosurveillance outbreak/epidemic, No traceability, No nais and beyond Washington, http://www.nonaiswa.org/?p=743.
2. Dictionary of Epidemiology 4th edn, 2001 John M Last.
3. Disease Outbreak Manual, Institute of Environmental Sciences and Research Limited, New Zealand, 2002. p. 97.
4. Endemic, Epidemic, Pandemic Epidemiology, http://en.wikipedia.org/wiki/endemic_.
5. Food-borne disease outbreaks-Guidelines for investigation and control-WHO 2008.
6. http://www.tsi.comuploadedFilesProduct_Information LiteratureApplication_NotesLC-105.pdf.
7. Infectious Disease Outbreak, Testimony before the Committee on Government Reform, April 9, 2003: Bioterrorism Preparedness Efforts have Improved Public Health Response Capacity, but Gaps Remain.
8. Influenza Pandemic Preparedness and Response Plan, Directorate General of Health Services, Ministry of Health and Family Welfare.www. http://mohfw.nic.in.
9. Mathur P. Hospital acquired infection: Prevention and control Wolters Khumer. Lippincott Williams and Wilkins, New Delhi 2010.
10. Model Plan for the management of communicable disease outbreaks in Wales. Welsh Collaboration on Health and Environment, March 1995.
11. National Centre for Disease Control, http://nicd.nic.in.
12. Park K Textbook of Preventive and Social Medicine, Banarsidas Bhanot, 20th edn, 2007.
13. Singh S, Gupta SK, Kant S. Hospital Infection Control Guidelines, Principles and Practices; Jaypee Brothers Medical Publishers, New Delhi, India, 2012.
14. UTAH Department of Health-Division of epidemiology and laboratory medicine.
15. WHO, Health topics-Disease outbreaks, http://www.who.int/topics/disease_outbreaks/en/.

16. WHO-Health Topics: International Health Regulations-Ports, Airports and Ground Crossings, http://www.who.int/ihr/ports_airports/en/.
17. WHO-Health Topics: International Health Regulations, http://www.who.int/topics/international_health_regulations/en/.
18. World Health Organizations-Areas of Work-Medicines-Pharmacovigilance, http://www.who.int/medicines/areas/quality_safety/...../index.

Index

V

W

Y